[

A beginners

MW01490687

By: Erik Smith

Table of Contents

Disclaimer

This document is geared towards providing exact and reliable information in regards to the topic and issue covered. The publication is sold with the idea that the publisher is not required to render accounting, officially permitted, or otherwise, qualified services. If advice is necessary, legal or professional, a practiced individual in the profession should be ordered.

- From a Declaration of Principles which was accepted and approved equally by a Committee of the American Bar Association and a Committee of Publishers and Associations.

The information herein is offered for informational purposes solely, and is universal as so. The presentation of the information is without contract or any type of guarantee assurance.

The trademarks that are used are without any consent, and the publication of the trademark is without permission or backing by the trademark owner. All trademarks and brands within this book are for

Free Bonus!

Do Want To Master your fitness and health so you can feel and look amazing in the next 60 days?

I have a free bonus for you that can help dramatically improve your health in fitness that I think you will like. I have put together a 5-Day email course that will help you look amazing, but more importantly you will also feel great as well.

If that's something you think you would like, sign up to get the emails starting today.

Sign up here - https://enlightenedmanuals.com/5-health-steps/

Free Books Every Week!

Do you want to get notified when I have free books? Then sign up for my newsletter. I will never spam you. I will only send you valuable stuff that you can use to help you improve your life.

Sign up here - https://enlightenedmanuals.com/free-books/

Introduction

I want to thank you and congratulate you for getting the book, "Dukan Diet."

As we all know, there are tons of dieting strategies out there these days and proponents of each proclaim that theirs is the most effective. While many of those diet regimens can help you shed those excess pounds, only a few can help you maintain your weight for life. The Dukan diet, dubbed as "the French solution to perpetual weight loss," will restructure your eating habits and with the goal of enabling you to maintain your weight for life without having to starve yourself.

Although it has faced several controversies since it was first developed, the Dukan diet is now one of the most (if not the most) popular diet methods of the modern day.

It currently has millions of advocates worldwide ranging from regular people to celebrities like Jessica Szohr and Jennifer Lopez and supermodels such as Gisele Bundchen.

The Dukan diet essentially consists of four phases—attack, cruise, consolidation and stabilization—to provide a more comprehensive approach not only to weight loss but to weight maintenance as well. This book will guide you through each phase and give you useful tips and information to help you achieve your weight loss goals.

Dieting does not need to mean starving --Many people struggling with weight problems will certainly appreciate that.

Thanks again for finding interest in this book. I hope you enjoy it!

What is the Dukan Diet?

The Dukan diet is a protein-based diet plan designed by French nutritionist and dietitian, Pierre Dukan. It is primarily intended as a rapid weight loss program that involves no counting of calories or feelings of hunger. However, your food choices are restricted to 100—of which 68 come from animal sources and 32 are plant-based. This means you can eat as much as you want, provided you stick to the list of 100 allowed foods.

The Promise

If you follow the rules of the Dukan diet, you could lose up to 10 pounds within one week and 2-4 pounds for each of the succeeding weeks until you reach your weight loss goal—all without utterly depriving yourself of food. If you continue to follow the diet rules up to the last phase, you will never gain those lost pounds back.

The Theory

The main focus of the Dukan diet is protein, which has low calorie content (only 4 calories per gram) compared to high-carb or high-fat foods. Protein also leaves a "satiating" effect so dieters tend to eat much less. And since the diet limits your consumption of carbs (the body's most preferred source of energy), your body is forced to burn fat stores as an alternative fuel, making you lose weight much quicker.

Dukan vs. Atkins

According to its proponents, the Dukan diet is similar to the Atkins diet in many ways. One of which is that both diets focus on low carb consumption in order to induce ketosis, a state wherein the body is prompted to burn fat for fuel, instead of sugar. However, these 2 diets also have some major differences:

·   Fat Content - the Dukan diet includes low-fat protein sources, whereas Atkins has no restriction on saturated fats (including meat fats) and dairy. Dr. Dukan proclaims that concentrating on low fat is better for heart health.

·   Natural Foods – the Dukan diet strictly implements the rule of sticking to the list of the 100 allowed foods, which are all 100% natural. On the other hand, the Atkins diet allows consumption of packaged foods, bars and shakes.

·   Calorie Counting – as previously mentioned, the Dukan diet does not involve calorie counting. Nor does it require counting other nutritional values during any of its 4 phases. The Atkins, however, restricts calorie intake during the entire course of the diet. That means you will have to count calories right from the beginning and for as long as you are on the diet.

·   Food Choices – the Atkins restricts vegetable consumption because dieters tend to go beyond their daily carb limit, whereas the Dukan diet allows you to eat vegetables as long as it is included in the list of allowed foods.

·   An Interactive, Personalized Diet Plan – the Dukan diet offers a personalized diet plan and features an online coaching support, which monitors the dieter's progress on a day-to-day basis. The Atkins diet has no similar program.

Note: This section does not intend to criticize the Atkins diet. It simply aims to describe the key differences between the two well-known diet methods to serve as a guide for dieters.

Your True Weight

Before starting the Dukan diet, it is essential to know your true weight first. Your true weight isn't necessarily the same as your desired or ideal weight. Rather, it is the realistic weight you can achieve without struggling or compromising your health. Also, it is the weight you're able to maintain long-term without difficulty, starvation and restricted food consumption.

Calculation of your true weight is available exclusively on the official website of the Dukan Diet. Once you're there, you will be asked to enter specific information into their online calculator. It will then create a personalized diet plan for you and determine your true weight goal. Required information includes the following:

·   age

·   gender

·   average weight

·   desired weight

·   lowest weight you have ever achieved

·   highest weight you have ever achieved

·   heredity (genetic trends in regards to weight gain)

·   number of pregnancies (if applicable)

·   bone structure

Based on the readings, the website will send you a graph and data demonstrating which phase of the Dukan diet you should be on and the length of time you should remain there.

Benefits of the Dukan Diet

The Dukan diet has been severely denounced by many nutritionists who regarded it as a dangerous restrictive diet. It was also criticized by the American Dietetic Association because it does not incorporate all the nutrients essential for good health. In spite of this, the Dukan diet certainly does what it's intended to do—to aid and sustain weight loss.

While there is not much research on the diet itself, the data concerning low-carb and low-fat diets are applicable to the Dukan method. In a study that compared the metabolic effects of a low-carb vs. a low-fat diet in obese and overweight subjects, the researchers found that the energy restriction attained by a low-carb diet is just as effective as a low-fat diet approach to fat-burning and weight loss. Since the Dukan diet is both low-carb and low-fat, the results of this study are as much valid for it. Below is a short list of the other health benefits that can be gained from following the Dukan approach.

· 	Reduces high blood pressure – a study indicates that low-carb and low-fat diets are equally effective to reduce diastolic blood pressure (by 5 mm. Hg) and systolic pressure (by 10 mm. Hg). This suggests that the diet may be useful in improving hypertension or high blood pressure.

· 	Reduces risk of cardiovascular disease - the same study points out that the LDL:HDL ratio, as well as the triglyceride:HDL ratio, were improved in both low-carb and low-carb diet strategy. This signifies that the Dukan diet may be beneficial in reducing risk factors of cardiovascular disease.

· 	Improves insulin sensitivity – although there are no scientific studies that demonstrate the direct connection between the Dukan diet and diabetes, researchers insinuate that losing weight generally helps improve insulin sensitivity, and in turn, improves type-2 diabetes. Low carb diets also aid the body to effectively break down fats, which are known to trigger insulin- related diseases.

In addition, the Dukan diet includes the following advantages:

·   You will lose a lot of weight during the initial phases of the Dukan diet. This is highly motivating for dieters and it encourages them to continue on with the diet.

·   The Dukan approach is easy to follow because you have a complete list of all the "allowed" and "not allowed" foods. You are also provided with an easy-to-understand diet plan so you'll know exactly on which phase you should be on.

·   Most diet methods will have you starving. With the Dukan diet, you can still enjoy food (only the allowed foods, of course). That means you will never have to endure hunger pangs. Additionally, protein is effective in satisfying hunger so you're less likely to feel hungry even while on the diet.

·   Since the diet cuts out foods that are high in fat and sugar, you are taking multiple steps away from obesity and other related complications.

·   There are various support groups and coaching programs that can be found on the internet and online forums. These can reduce boredom and help with encouragement while you're on the diet.

·   As a member of the Dukan personalized weight-loss coaching (on Dukan diet official website), you have exclusive and unlimited access to the 100 allowed foods and valuable information about their nutritional qualities and properties. You can also check the list of the tolerated foods and foods that leave a satiating (full) effect. If you have run out of recipe ideas, there are tons of Dukan diet recipes available, as well as food tips to help you maximize your success on the program.

But as with all diet techniques, the Dukan diet also has some drawbacks. Since it disregards key principles of healthy eating,—such as the importance of fruits, the benefits of fiber and whole grains, and the advantages of selecting from a wide array of food choices—this diet has the tendency to be nutritionally imbalanced. Consequently, people who follow the Dukan approach or any other type of low-carb diet may experience the following side-effects:

· Lack of energy – due to low levels of carbohydrates, you may experience lethargy and nausea which may affect your physical and mental functions.

· Digestion issues – due to inadequate levels of fiber in your body, diarrhea, constipation, irritable bowel syndrome (IBS) and other digestive problems may be triggered.

· Impaired kidney function – high protein, low-carb diets have a direct link to kidney functions and may create potential risks of kidney diseases.

· Increased risk of osteoporosis – since high-protein diets require processing of more calcium, your body will start extracting the required amount of calcium from your bones. This may lead to bone density loss which may result in osteoporosis in the long run. You can manage this by eating more calcium-rich food or taking calcium supplements.

· Nutrient deficiencies – due to the restricted food choice—which mainly includes high protein, low carbohydrates, low fat and no fiber— there is a deficiency of the required daily amount of certain nutrients, such as Vitamins B and E.

Bad breath, dry mouth, frequent urination and irritability are other possible side-effects of the Dukan diet.

Important Reminder

The Dukan diet results in weight/fat loss which is usually beneficial for many common health conditions. In certain cases, however, the benefits of the diet may be outweighed by the risks.

If you are on medication for diabetes, your dose likely needs to be adjusted. If you suffer from renal disease, your kidneys may be loaded with more protein than they can handle. And if you have any type of heart disease, you would miss out on heart-healthy fibers if you followed the Dukan diet. This diet may also be unsafe for individuals at risk of electrolyte imbalance. Due to the restrictive nature of the Dukan method, it is important to talk to your doctor first before switching to this new diet plan.

The Four Phases

The Dukan diet consists of four phases. The first two phases concentrate on high-protein, low-fat and low-carb foods, while the final two phases have to do with reintroduction of foods, which aims to help dieters maintain their newly-achieved weight.

1: Attack Phase

The Attack phase involves pure protein and can last between 5-10 days depending on your weight goal. The main objective here is to lose weight fast – usually 4-7 pounds in five days. During this phase, you are allowed to eat 68 protein-rich foods that can produce noticeable and immediate weight loss results. The Attack phase is also a way to kick-start your metabolism. Below is the list of the 68 protein food sources that you can eat during this phase.

68 Protein-Rich Foods:

·   Dairy Products

cottage cheese, cream cheese, milk, plain Greek yogurt, ricotta, sour cream

*Always buy fat-free dairy products.

·   Eggs

chicken eggs – duck eggs – quail eggs

·   Fish & Shellfish

arctic char – catfish – clams – cod – crab – crawfish/crayfish – flounder – freshwater trout – grouper – haddock – halibut/smoked halibut – herring – lobster – mackerel – mahi mahi – monk fish – mussels – octopus – orange roughy – oysters – perch – red snapper – salmon/smoked salmon

– sardines (canned or fresh) – scallops – sea bass – shark – shrimp – sole – squid – surimi – sword fish – tilapia – tuna (canned or fresh)

- Lean Meat

beef tenderloin – buffalo – deer meat (venison) – extra lean ham – extra lean kosher beef hotdogs – filet mignon – flank steak – lean pork chops (center-cut) – London broil steak – low-fat bacon/soy bacon – pork tenderloin – roast beef (lean slices) – roast pork loin – sirloin steak– veal chops – veal scaloppini

- Poultry Products

chicken – chicken/turkey sausage (fat-free) – chicken liver – Cornish hen – low-fat deli slices of turkey or chicken – ostrich steak – quail – turkey meat – wild duck

- Vegetarian Proteins

seitan – soy foods – tempeh – tofu – veggie burgers

2: Cruise Phase

During this phase, carbohydrates are gradually reintroduced with the addition of 32 non-starchy vegetables (fruits are strictly not allowed). You will now have a total of 100 foods to choose from. You can alternate pure-protein days and protein-plus-vegetables days to promote a steady weight loss. This phase can last for a few months (3 days for every pound you want to shed). The vegetables allowed during the Cruise phase are as follows.

32 Vegetables:

artichoke – arugula/lettuce/radicchio – asparagus – bean sprouts – bell peppers – beets – broccoli – Brussels sprouts – cabbages – carrots – cauliflower – celery sticks – cucumber – eggplant – endives – fennels – green beans – kale – leeks/onions/shallots – mushrooms – okra – palm hearts – pumpkin – radish – rhubarb – spaghetti squash – spinach – squash – tomatoes – turnip – water cress – zucchini

3: Consolidation Phase

The consolidation phase is purported to prevent your body from gaining back the weight it has lost. This is done by gradually returning foods that were previously forbidden. You can still eat unlimited protein and vegetables every day, with the addition of 1 piece of low-carb fruit, 2 healthy slices of whole grain bread and 1 small serving of cheese. Every week, you can also enjoy 2 "celebration" meals wherein you can eat whatever food you want.

The consolidation phase has a strict timeline that should be followed: 5 days for each pound you lost in the Cruise phase. It is also essential to follow one more important rule: to have a pure-protein day each week (preferably the same day every week).

4: Stabilization Phase

The final phase is all about weight maintenance and should be followed for the rest of your life. Only a few rules are involved here: eat 3 tbsp. of oat bran every day, have a pure-protein day every week, take a 20-minute-walk daily and take the stairs instead of elevators and escalators (whenever possible).

The stabilization phase must be incorporated into your lifestyle in order to keep the weight off permanently. Since you have learned the right approach to healthy eating and established a pattern, it is now easier to maintain your new lean body. Commitment is the key.

The Secret Ingredient

One of the key elements that differentiate the Dukan diet from other no-carb diet regimens is oat bran. It is rich in soluble fiber and protein and helps you feel full because it expands up to 20x its size in your stomach. It is also good for the heart and eases constipation, bloating and other problems with digestion.

Although it's not on the list, oat bran should be included in your diet every day (as recommended by Dr. Dukan). You can eat 1.5 tablespoons of oat bran per day during the attack phase and 2 tablespoons during the cruise and consolidation phase.

What to Drink

Staying hydrated is vital when you're on a diet (and even when you're not), so always ensure you get the right amount of fluids every day.

· Water – tap, bottled or sparkling

· Tea – sugar-free; but you can add skimmed milk or diet-friendly sweeteners

· Any other non-caloric drinks – avoid carbonated and energy drinks (even the ones labeled "sugar-free" or "low-carb") as they are often packed with sugar.

Additional Foods Allowed on the Diet

· Olive oil – You can use limited amount (1 tsp.) of olive oil beginning from the Cruise up to the last phase. Olive oil is rich in Vitamin E, polyphenols and omega-3 fatty acids—all of which are vital for good health.

· Goji berries – You can eat limited quantity of Goji berries starting from the first phase. Recommended amount is 1 tbsp. on pure-protein days and 2 tbsp. on proteins + vegetables days. Tablespoons shouldn't be heaping.

· Shirataki – You can eat as much Shirataki as you'd like starting from the first phase. The Asian Konjac root is rich in fiber and has almost no calories. It also keeps you feeling full and promotes proper intestinal transit. Besides its raw form, Konjac is also available in powder form (flour) and occasionally in gel form.

The Dukan diet doesn't promise extreme weight loss results by end of the first 3 phases. Rather, it guarantees that if you strictly follow the rules, you will achieve your true weight goal and maintain it for life.

Diet Tips and Friendly Reminders

The Dukan diet is not something you can bite off thoughtlessly and spit out when you realize it's more than you can chew. Although it does not restrict how much you can eat, it does restrict what you can eat. As this world is full of temptations, serious amount of self-control and discipline is required. Before you get started with the Dukan diet, here are 7 important steps that warrant your consideration:

1.   Find your true weight – This determines your overall weight goal and creates your personalized program, including the duration and your weight loss goal for each of the 3 initial phases.

2.   List all your motivations for losing weight – This will help you stick to the challenge and achieve your goals.

3.   Talk to your doctor – Your doctor will do an initial check-up (stress test, blood pressure, blood work, etc.) to ensure you're fit before you start the diet. He/she will also give you constructive advices to make the program a success.

4.   Talk to your family and friends – Your family and friends are your best allies during the entire weight loss program. Let them know that their support is extremely important and will be greatly appreciated. You can also interact with the other members of the community and participate in online forums by joining the coaching program on DukanDiet.com.

5.   Choose a start date – This will set you on the right track towards change and weight loss.

6.   Stock up on with the allowed foods and eliminate all temptations – Sort through your fridge, cupboards and pantry and replace all the "forbidden" foods with the 100 allowed foods.

7.   Choose how you want to stay on the Dukan diet – you may follow the diet alone, with the help of a Dukan book, with close family members or friends, with the Dukan diet community or with the official coaching program on the Dukan diet website.

Once you have accomplished these 7 steps, then you're ready to start the Dukan diet and begin the Attack phase. Apparently though, many Dukan dieters (or "Dukanians," as they are called) struggle in the middle of the diet and experience some setbacks. If you find yourself facing a problem, here are 10 additional tips and advices to get you back on track.

1.   Build a support system – Whenever you feel like giving up on the diet, turn to your spouse/partner, colleagues, friends and online communities and seek support. Most often than not, they will give you compliments and moral support which will give more motivation and strength to continue on. If you think that you're doing this not only for yourself but for others well, giving up will never be an option.

2.   Exercise – This is an essential component of any weight loss approach. Lack of physical activity while dieting can negatively affect your metabolism and slow down your progress. When you exercise and raise your heart rate, you will notice positive changes within 3-4 days. It does not need to be a vigorous exercise. You can simply have a run or perform a low-intensity workout. That is enough to boost your metabolism and accelerate your progress.

3.   Don't cheat – Cheating on a diet is the riskiest thing you can ever do. Once you chomp on a forbidden food, you may not want to stop and that will ruin the entire thing. Everything thereafter becomes multiple times harder. Here are two tips to avoid cheating and temptations altogether: (1) Always have diet-friendly snacks available (pickles, celery sticks, low-carb smoothies, oat bran, etc.) so when the hunger pang attacks, you can quickly and easily curb it and forget about your cravings. (2) Shop for grocery on a full stomach, so you will not be tempted to throw in prohibited foods in your cart and have a supply of them in your kitchen.

4.   Track your progress – Weighing yourself every day and constantly seeing a drop on the scale is the easiest way to stay motivated. However, don't always keep your hopes exceedingly high. There may be some

days when you see little or no improvement but that does not mean your efforts are fruitless. Keep a record of your progress on a daily basis and always look at the bigger picture. If necessary, search for the reasons why you can't shed additional weight. The solution is usually handy and you don't always need to start from scratch.

5.   Plan your meals in advance – This is a good way to avoid dropping by the fast food drive-through or calling for pizza delivery. Having a meal plan is almost always necessary when you're on a diet as it keeps everything organized and prevents you from giving into your cravings.

6.   Don't party on an empty stomach – Just because you're on a diet doesn't mean you have to give up your social life. You can still go to parties and attend social gatherings—just not on an empty stomach. By going to the party with a full belly, you can save yourself from the trouble of overeating once you're there. If possible, have a seat somewhere distant from the buffet table. Drink water and chew some sugar-free gum to keep your mouth occupied.

7.   Avoid "risky" situations – While some social events are easy to get through, some are just too risky. Bar nights and all-you-can-eat get-togethers are one of those situations wherein it's too tempting not to cheat on your diet. In cases like these, don't be afraid to say no. Assess the circumstances first and if you can't say no, then simply don't go.

8.   Set realistic goals – If you set goals like "lose 5 pounds overnight" or "lose 50 pounds in one month," you will feel further away from your weight loss goals which will consequently make you feel more discouraged. Break those big goals into small, achievable ones and you will feel more stimulated once you have achieved them.

9.   Commit – Do not attempt to go on a restrictive diet if your whole heart is not into it. That is the quickest way to sabotage the diet completely. If you're not committed, you're likely to give into the very first temptation and cheat every time cheating is called for. Before you begin any type of diet, make sure both your mind and body are seriously prepared.

10.   Reward yourself – Not with cheating on the diet but with something that you will appreciate and can benefit from. Small things will do like treating yourself to a massage or buying that pair of shoes you've been eyeing up. Rewarding yourself every time you've accomplished a small goal is another way to keep yourself motivated.

There may be many obstacles towards the success of the Dukan diet, but there are even more resolutions that can negate them. The most important of all is to always stay motivated. Always remind yourself of your goals and think of those people who are rooting for you. It may be a tough ride, but it's definitely a rewarding one as well.

15 Simple Dukan Diet Recipes

Although the Dukan menu includes limited amount of ingredients, you can still enjoy varied meals every day. Provided below are 15 Dukan recipes—5 of which focus on protein, 5 on vegetables and the other 5 are smoothies and oat bran recipes. These are all easy to follow and everyone can do these recipes at home.

Protein Recipes

Beef Kebabs

Ingredients:

1 tbsp cider vinegar

2 tbsp mild mustard

1 bay leaf

50ml low-sodium soy sauce

Small amount of thyme

Vegetable oil

50ml lemon juice

400g beef fillet (large chunks)

Instructions:

1.   Combine all the ingredients and marinate in the refrigerator for 2-4 hours.

2.   Remove the marinade.

3.   Place the beef chunks on the skewers and grill until cooked.

Salmon with Ginger

Ingredients:

2 garlic gloves

1 salmon fillet

50ml low-sodium soy sauce

50ml teriyaki sauce

Ginger to taste

Instructions:

1.   Preheat the oven to 250° C.

2.   Put the salmon in a foil on a baking dish.

3.   Seal the foil on each side and leave a small space inside it to allow for circulation of hot air.

4.   Bake for 15 minutes.

Shrimps in Herbs

Ingredients:

900g shrimps (skinned, deveined and rinsed)

4 garlic cloves (minced)

30g fresh parsley

50ml dry white wine

1 fresh lemon (sliced in half)

Instructions:

1.   In a frying pan, combine the shrimps, garlic and parsley.

2.   Add wine and sauté until the shrimps turn pink.

3.   Serve with lemon.

Tandoori Chicken Escalopes

Ingredients:

3 garlic cloves

2 green chilies

2cm-piece ginger

Salt & pepper

2 pots of non-fat yogurt

2 tbsp tandoori-masala spice

6 chicken breast fillets

Fresh lemon juice

Instructions:

1.   Combine all the ingredients, except chicken meat.

2.   Crush the garlic, chilies, ginger and other spices to completion.

3.   Score the fillets so that the spice-yogurt mixture seeps into the meat.

4.   Marinate the chicken overnight in the refrigerator.

5.   The following day, cook the marinated chicken for 20 minutes in an oven preheated to 200° C.

6.   Remove the chicken from the oven and grill (until it turns brown or cooked to your liking) before serving.

Cottage Cheese Jelly

Ingredients:

355ml boiling water

250g fat-free cottage cheese

9g jelly lite

Instructions:

1.	Put the jelly in a bowl of boiling water and mix until dissolved.

2.	Work the cottage cheese in a blender until smooth.

3.	Combine jelly and cottage cheese then pour the creamy mixture into small cups or a bowl.

4.	Refrigerate until the mixture set.

Vegetable Recipes

Kale Crisps

Ingredients:

1 head of kale

2 tbsp olive oil

A sprinkle of sea salt

Instructions:

1.	Preheat the oven to 135° C.

2.	Rip the kale into tiny pieces.

3.	Mix with salt and oil and spread evenly on a baking tray.

4.	Bake for about 20 minutes or until crisp.

Stuffed Mushrooms

Ingredients:

2 garlic cloves

30g fresh parsley

A few teaspoons of skim milk

Small drops of vegetable oil

20 large mushrooms

Salt and pepper to taste

Instructions:

1.   Preheat the oven to 200° C.

2.   Wash the mushrooms and take out the stalks.

3.   Chop the stalks and add all the other ingredients. This will be the stuffing mixture.

4.   Cook the mixture in a frying pan until done.

5.   Meanwhile, place the mushroom caps (cap side up) on a baking tray and bake for 10 minutes.

6.   Fill the caps of the mushrooms with the stuffing mixture and bake for another 20 minutes.

7.   When done, drizzle a few drops of vegetable oil over the stuffed mushrooms and serve.

Broccoli-Bacon Mozzarella Bake

Ingredients:

750g broccoli

50ml low-fat chicken broth

1 tbsp Italian seasoning

125g FF Mozzarella

100g low-fat bacon

1 teaspoon paprika spice

Salt & pepper

Instructions:

1.   Preheat your oven to 350° F.

2.   Boil the broccoli in the chicken broth until it softens.

3.   Put the broccoli on a baking tray and pour in the chicken broth.

4.   Cut thin slices of the FF mozzarella cheese and place them on the broccoli.

5.   Scatter low-fat bacon cubes and sprinkle the seasoning and spices to taste.

6.   Bake for 20 minutes.

Cabbage Hamburgers

Ingredients:

5g baking powder

6 tbsp corn flour

1 onion (chopped)

1 large yellow onion

3 eggs

6 tbsp oat bran

500g cabbage (finely chopped/shredded)

Instructions:

1.   Mix all the ingredients together.

2.   Cook in a frying pan or bake in the oven at 180° C.

Stuffed Spicy Cucumbers

Ingredients:

1 garlic clove

2 cucumbers

¾ cup fat-free Greek yogurt

Instructions:

1.   Mix garlic, yogurt and spices together.

2.   Remove the center of the cucumbers.

3.   Stuff the garlic-yogurt mixture into the cucumber slices and serve.

Oat Bran & Smoothies

Oat Bran Granola

Ingredients:

2 tbsp oat bran

1 tbsp sugar-free syrup

Instructions:

1.   Mix the syrup and oat bran together in a microwavable bowl.

2.   Cook in a microwave for 1 ½ minutes.

3.   Let cool and serve with fat-free yogurt.

Zucchini Oat Bran Muffins

Ingredients:

1 teaspoon baking soda

1 tbsp low-fat cocoa powder (unsweetened)

½ cup fat-free milk

1/3 cup fat-free Greek yogurt

3 large eggs

1.5 cups oat bran

1 tbsp pumpkin spice

1 cup Splenda

1 tbsp vanilla extract

1 cup fresh zucchini (shredded, with juice)

Instructions:

1.   Mix dry and wet ingredients in two separate bowls.

2.   Combine dry to wet mixture gradually, stirring with a spoon while you do so.

3.   Line a muffin sheet with thin paper cups and pour the mixture into the cups evenly.

4.   Bake for 20 minutes.

Petits Pains D'Avoine

Ingredients:

1 teaspoon baking powder

2 tbsp fat-free cottage cheese

2 eggs

2 tbsp oat bran

1 teaspoon salt

4 tbsp fat-free yogurt

Instructions:

1. Preheat the oven to 200° C.

2. Combine all ingredients until smooth.

3. Pour the mixture into a baking plate designed to make small bread shape.

4. Bake for 25 minutes.

Blueberry Kale Smoothie

Ingredients:

1 tbsp almond butter

1 cup frozen blueberries

½ cup ice

½ cup kale

½ cup non-fat vanilla yogurt

Ingredients:

1. Add all the ingredients into a blender.

2. Blend to smoothness and pour into a tall cup.

Lean Green Protein Smoothie

Ingredients:

½ celery stalk

1 tbsp chia seeds

1 cup cold water

1 tbsp flaxseed oil

1 packet dried wheatgrass

1 cup frozen spinach

½ cup frozen broccoli

1 cup kale

Instructions:

1.   Mix all the ingredients in a blender.

2.   Blend to smoothness and serve.

Feel free to adjust the ingredients if there are food items you're allergic to or simply don't like. As mentioned, there are hundreds more Dukan diet recipes online so you don't need to repeat recipes and bore yourself. If you feel hungry between main meals, remember you can always grab a snack from the list of allowed foods. There is absolutely no need to endure your hunger—that's one of the best things about the Dukan diet.

Conclusion

Thank you again for getting this book!

I hope you found valuable information from this book and ample encouragement to get started on the Dukan diet. Although it was initially deemed ineffective (without strong scientific basis) by many dietitians and health experts, the Dukan diet is now proven effective with millions of people on its defense.

There are also many general practitioners and nutritionists who recommend the diet to many of their patients as they believe in its efficacy in stabilizing weight in the long term. With those said, there is virtually no reason not to try the Dukan diet today. This isn't only for weight loss per se, but for the betterment of your general health as well.

Thank you and good luck!

Free Bonus!

Do Want To Master your fitness and health so you can feel and look amazing in the next 60 days?

I have a free bonus for you that can help dramatically improve your health in fitness that I think you will like. I have put together a 5-Day email course that will help you look amazing, but more importantly you will also feel great as well.

If that's something you think you would like, sign up to get the emails starting today.

Sign up here - https://enlightenedmanuals.com/5-health-steps/

Free Books Every Week!

Do you want to get notified when I have free books? Then sign up for my newsletter. I will never spam you. I will only send you valuable stuff that you can use to help you improve your life.

Sign up here - https://enlightenedmanuals.com/free-books/

Made in United States
Orlando, FL
29 April 2025